OXFORD GENERAL PRACTICE LIBRARY

Pain and Palliation

Dr Max Watson

Lecturer, Palliative Medicine,
University of Ulster,
Honorary Consultant Palliative Medicine,
Northern Ireland Hospice,
Belfast, and Princess Alice Hospice,
Esher, and Clinical Adviser,
Hospice Friendly Hospitals Program,
Dublin.

Dr Karen O'Reilly

General Practitioner, Bishops Waltham,
Hampshire.

Dr Chantal Simon

General Practitioner, Bournemouth,
Dorset, and Editor of InnovAiT.

and Series Editor

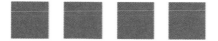

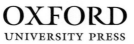

OXFORD
UNIVERSITY PRESS

OXFORD
UNIVERSITY PRESS

Great Clarendon Street, Oxford OX2 6DP

Oxford University Press is a department of the University of Oxford.
It furthers the University's objective of excellence in research, scholarship,
and education by publishing worldwide in

Oxford New York

Auckland Cape Town Dar es Salaam Hong Kong Karachi
Kuala Lumpur Madrid Melbourne Mexico City Nairobi
New Delhi Shanghai Taipei Toronto

With offices in

Argentina Austria Brazil Chile Czech Republic France Greece
Guatemala Hungary Italy Japan Poland Portugal Singapore
South Korea Switzerland Thailand Turkey Ukraine Vietnam

Oxford is a registered trade mark of Oxford University Press
in the UK and in certain other countries

Published in the United States
by Oxford University Press, Inc., New York

British Library Cataloguing in Publication Data
Data available

Library of Congress Cataloging in Publication Data
Data available

Typeset by Newgen Imaging Systems (P) Ltd., Chennai, India
Printed in Great Britain
on acid-free paper by
Ashford Colour Press Ltd., Gosport, Hampshire.

ISBN 978–0–19–921572–0

10 9 8 7 6 5 4 3 2 1